C000119083

# You Are So Much More

## An Inspiration for Children
## Healing From Illness or Injury

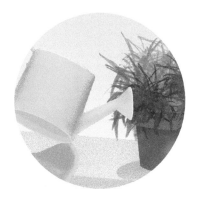

BY SERENA TEJPAR

*Illustrated by Anoosha Lalani and Iman Tejpar*

# You Are So Much More

## By Serena Tejpar

Copyright © Loving Healing Press

Library of Congress Cataloging-in-Publication Data

| | |
|---|---|
| Publisher: | Loving Healing Press |
| Author: | Serena Tejpar |
| Illustrator: | Anoosha Lalani & Iman Tejpar |
| ISBN-13: | PB 978-1-61599-632-2 / HC 978-161599-633-9 / eBook 978-1-61599-634-6 |
| List Price: | PB $ 16.95 / HC $ 28.95 / eBook $ 4.95 |
| Audio-book: | iTunes, Audible.com, Amazon |
| Trim: | 8.5 x 8.5 (44 pp) |
| Audience: | 5-7 years |
| Pub Date: | 06/01/2022 |
| BISAC: | Juvenile Fiction/Health & Daily Living/Diseases, Illnesses & Injuries |
| | Juvenile Fiction/Social Issues/Self-Esteem & Self-Reliance |
| | Juvenile Fiction/Social Issues/Emotions & Feel-ings |
| Distributor: | Ingram (USA/CAN/AU), Bertram's Books (UK/EU) |

No part of this publication may be reproduced or distributed in any
form or by any means, or stored in a database or retrieval system,
without the prior written permission of the publisher.

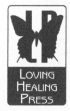

Published by:
Loving Healing Press
5145 Pontiac Trail
Ann Arbor, MI 48105
USA
Website: www.LHPress.com
Email:info@LHPress.com
Toll-free: 888-761-6268
Fax: 734-663-6861

# Dedication

To all those young children sleeping in hospital beds with acute illnesses and chronic conditions waiting for the moment they can run through the playground and just be a kid again—remember that there is so much more to you.

# Acknowledgment

I would like to express my sincere gratitude to my aunt and second mom, Shaila Abdullah, an accomplished author, who has always nurtured my creativity and encouraged me to put pen to paper and share my story.

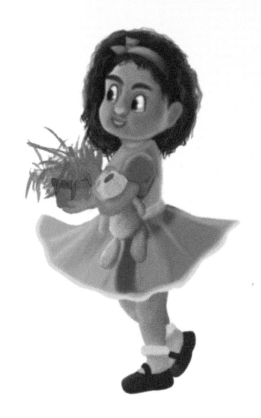

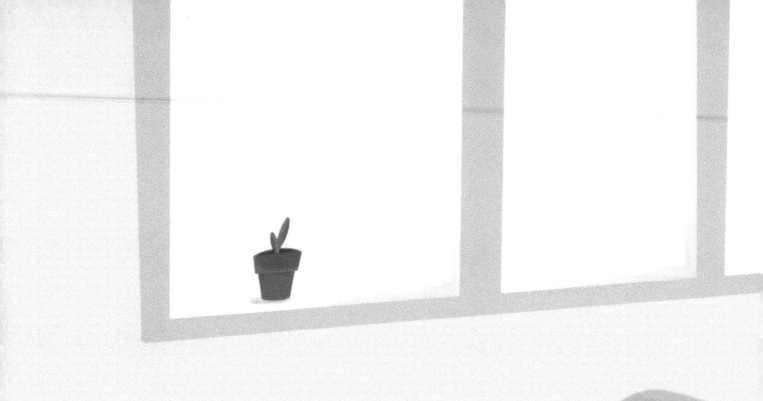

When you are sitting in that hospital bed feeling

**Oh-so-crummy**

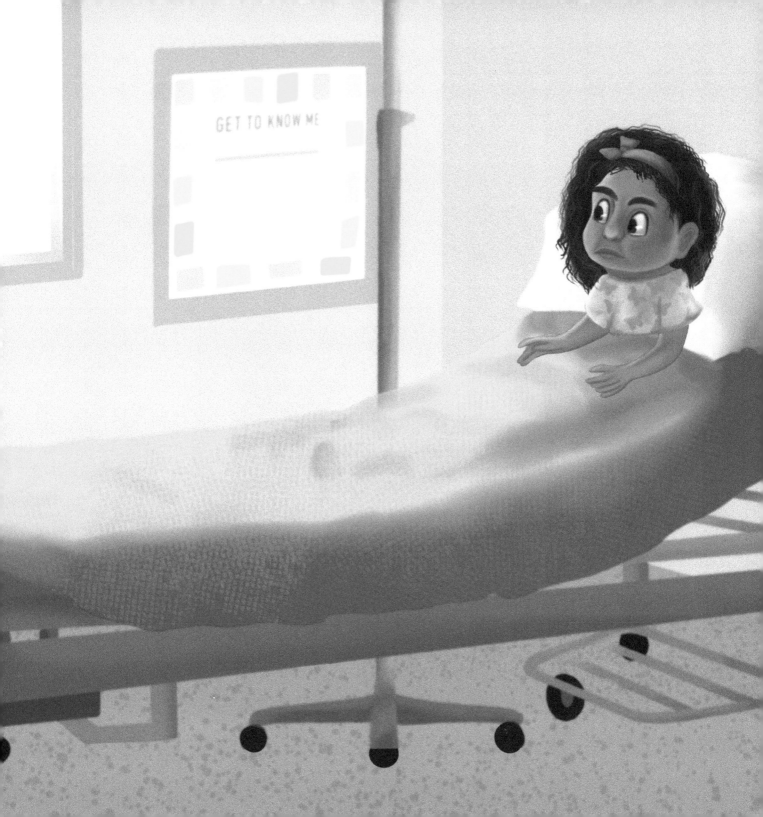

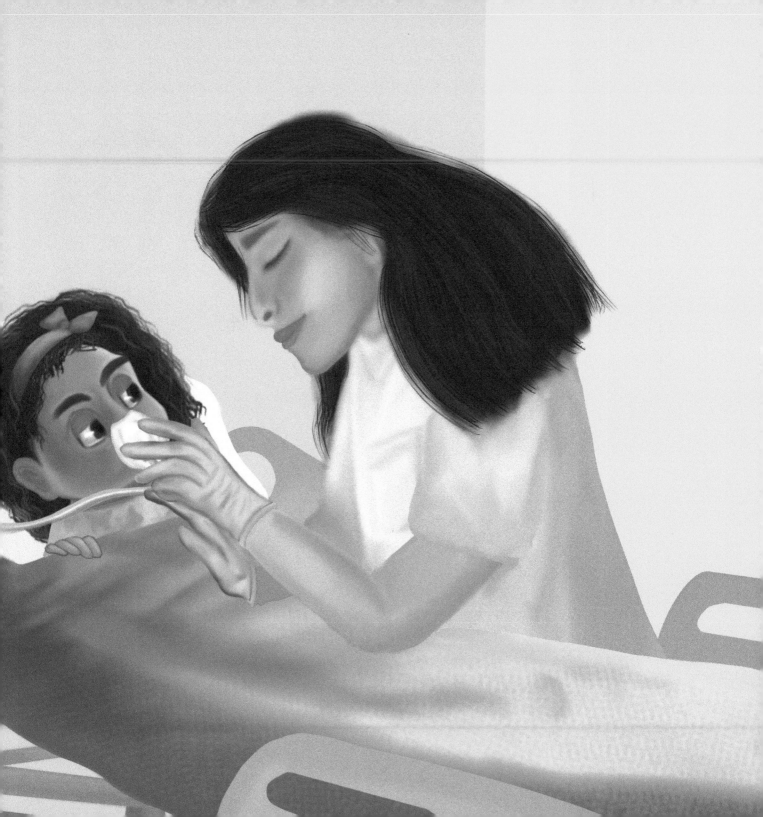

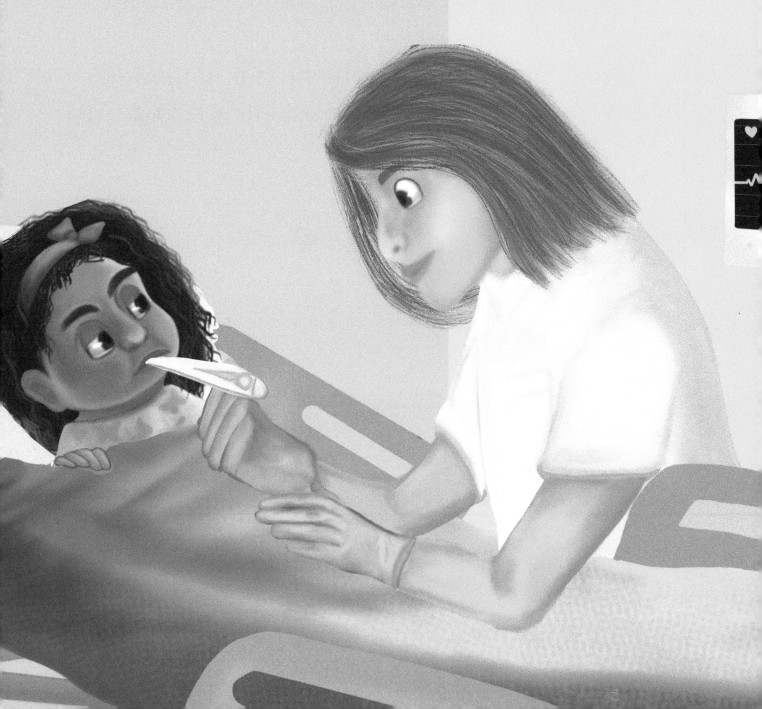

with doctors and nurses coming and going

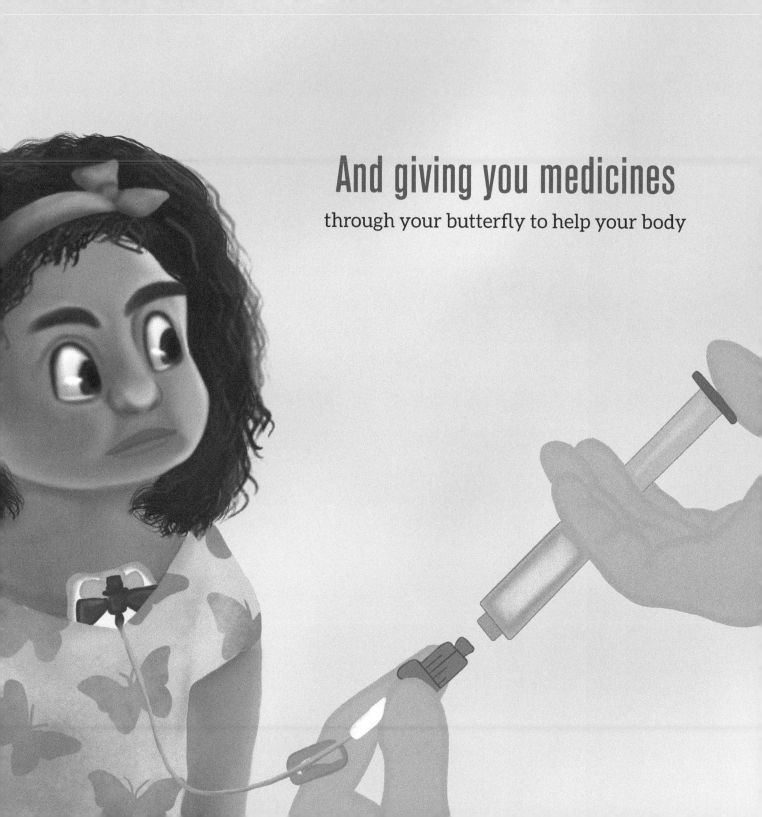

# And giving you medicines

through your butterfly to help your body

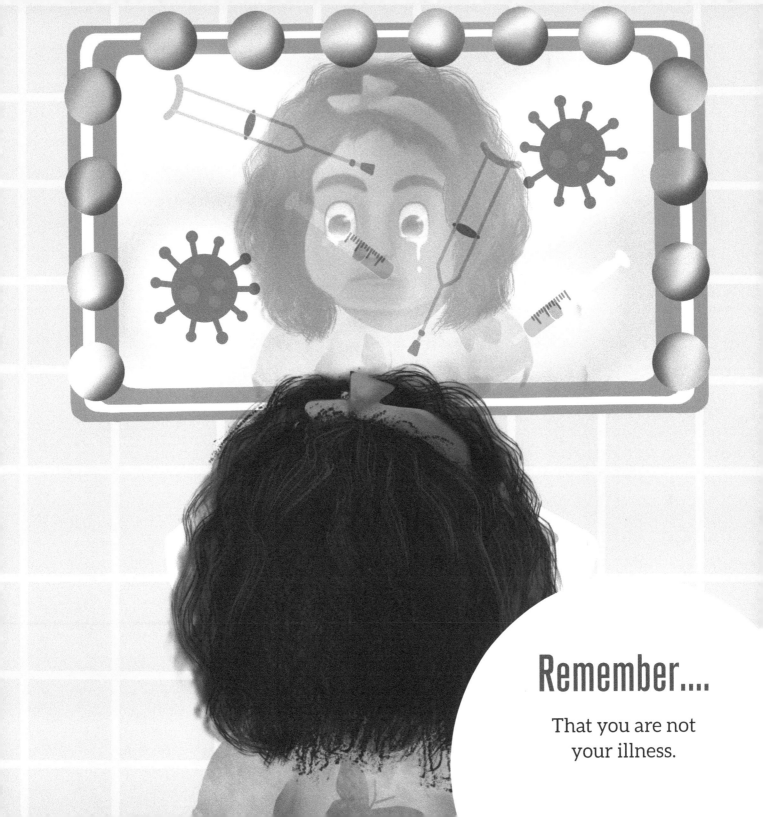

Remember....

That you are not
your illness.

# You are far more

### than the medicines you take,

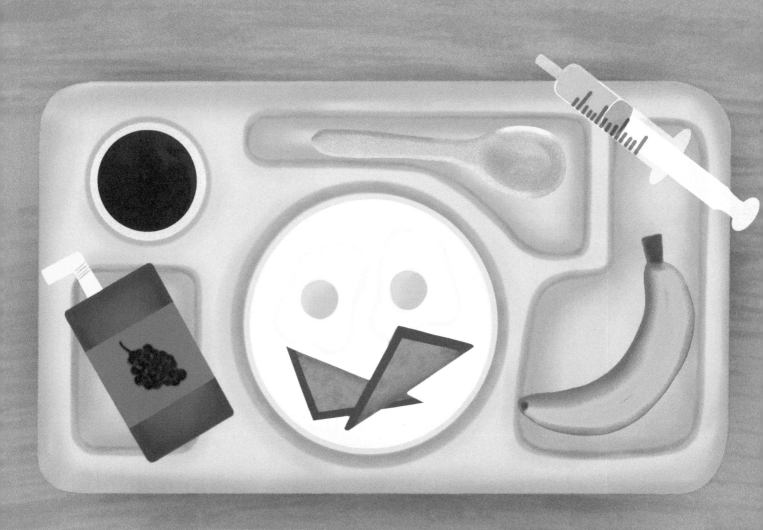

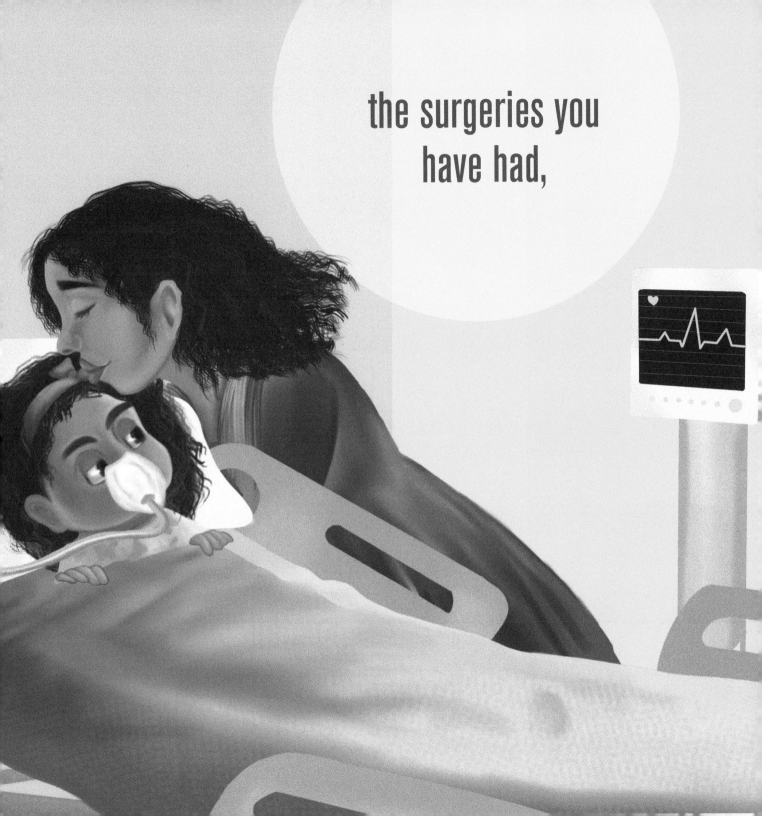

the surgeries you
have had,

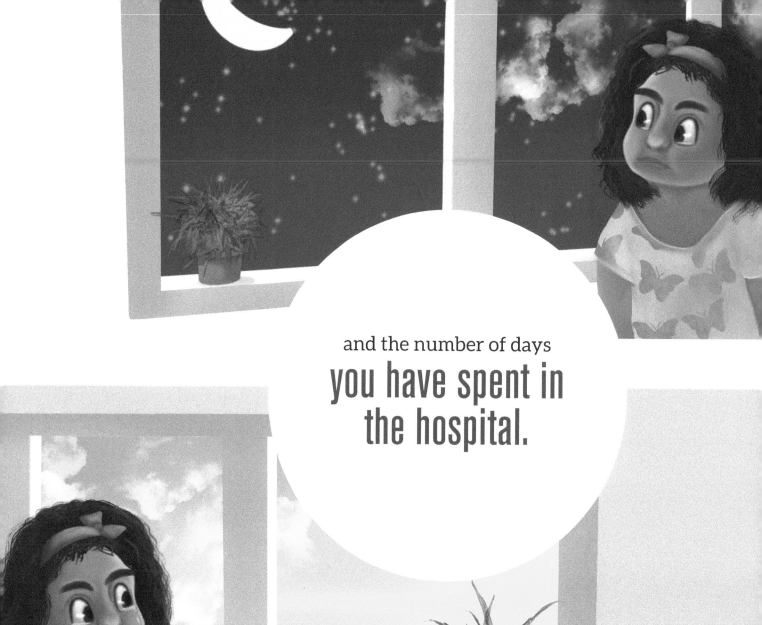

and the number of days
you have spent in
the hospital.

You are **SO** much more than that.

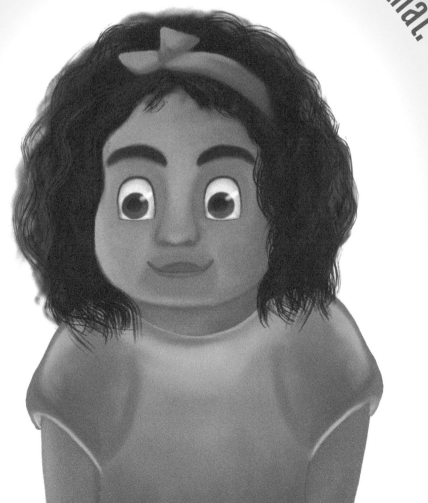

You are a loving soul.
A child.
A little giggler.
An explorer.
A friend.
The most mischievous little munchkin.

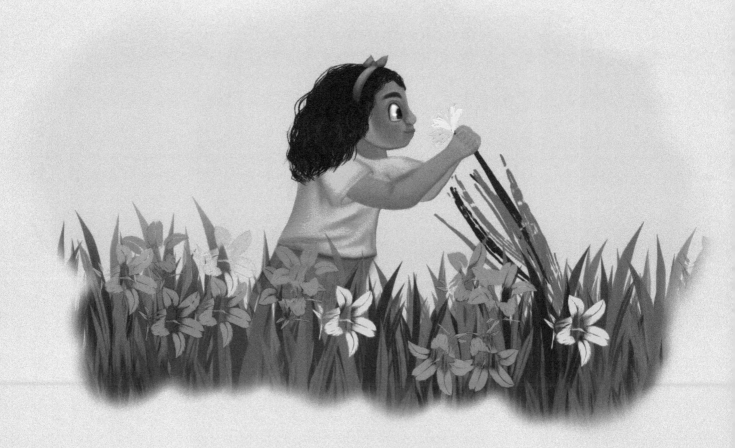

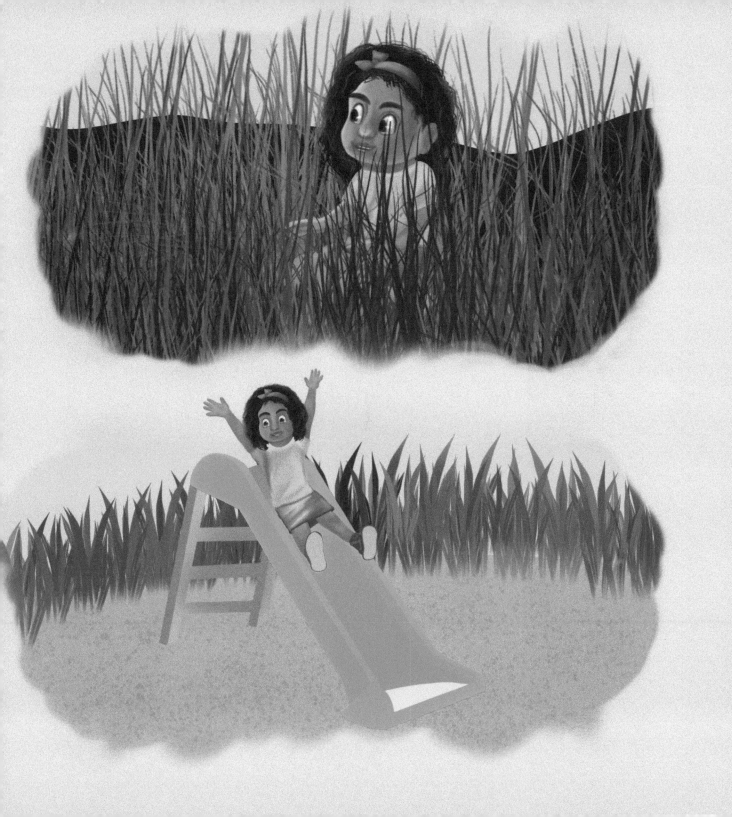

# You are brave.

Facing every challenge,
every fear, one step at a time.

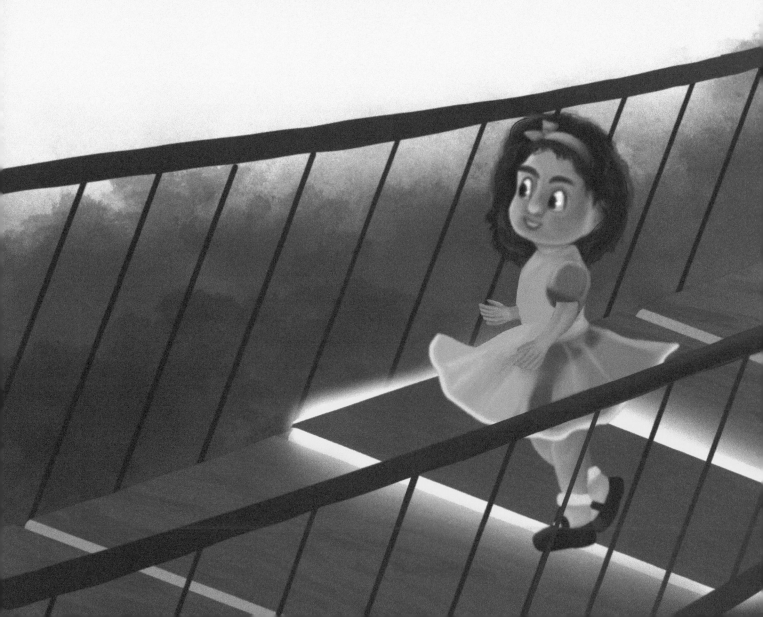

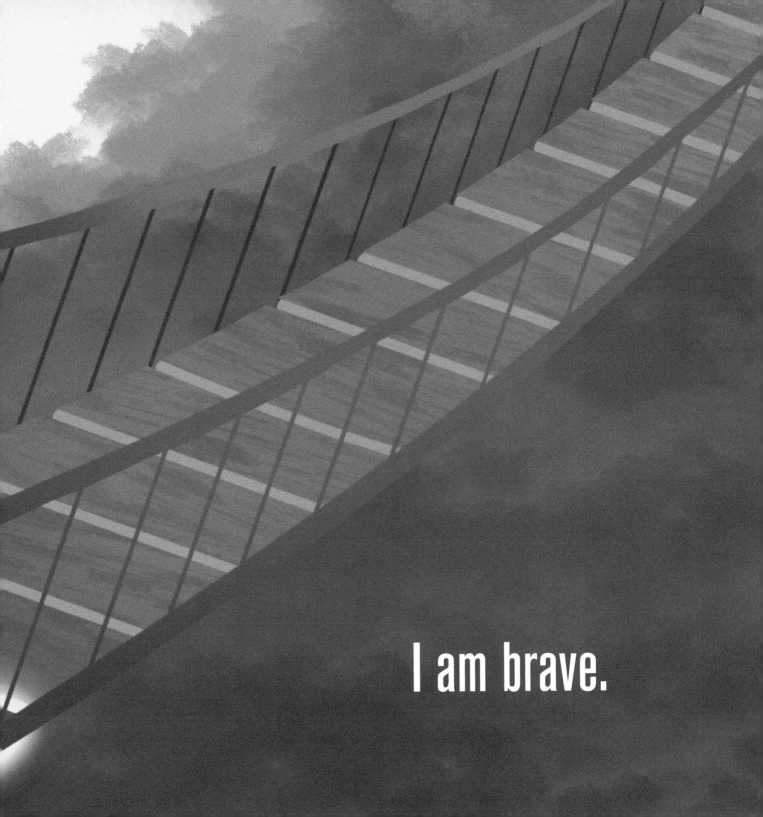

I am brave.

# You are strong.

Your journey has not been easy, and your path may feel topsy-turvy. It's okay to cry, your tears show your strength.

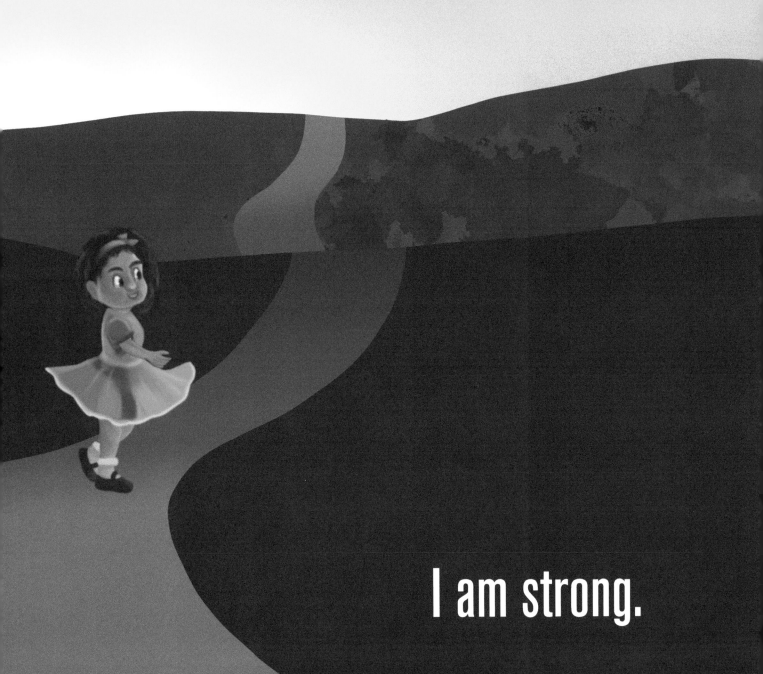

I am strong.

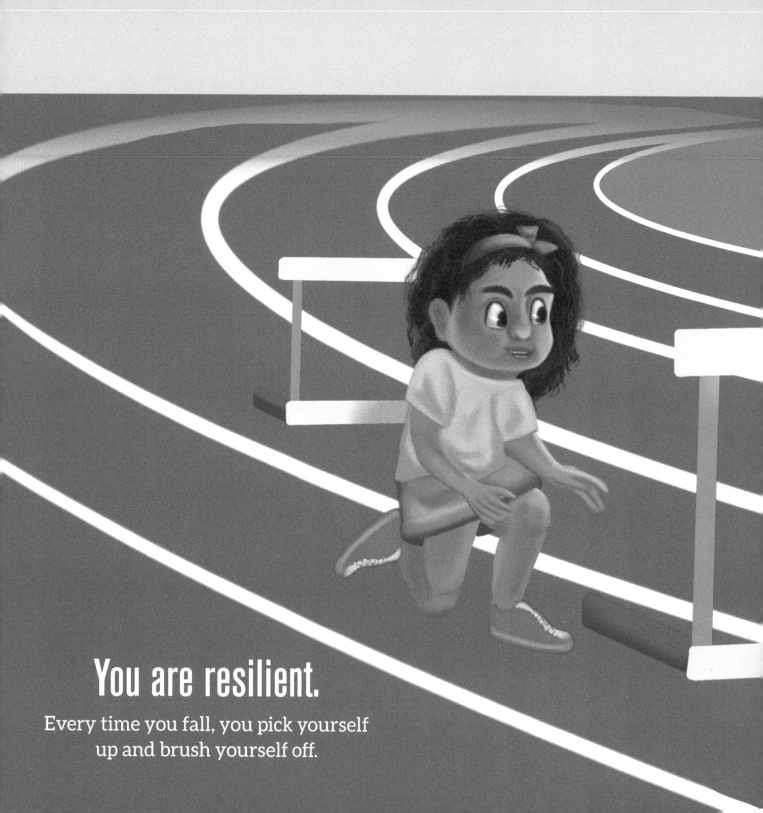

# You are resilient.

Every time you fall, you pick yourself
up and brush yourself off.

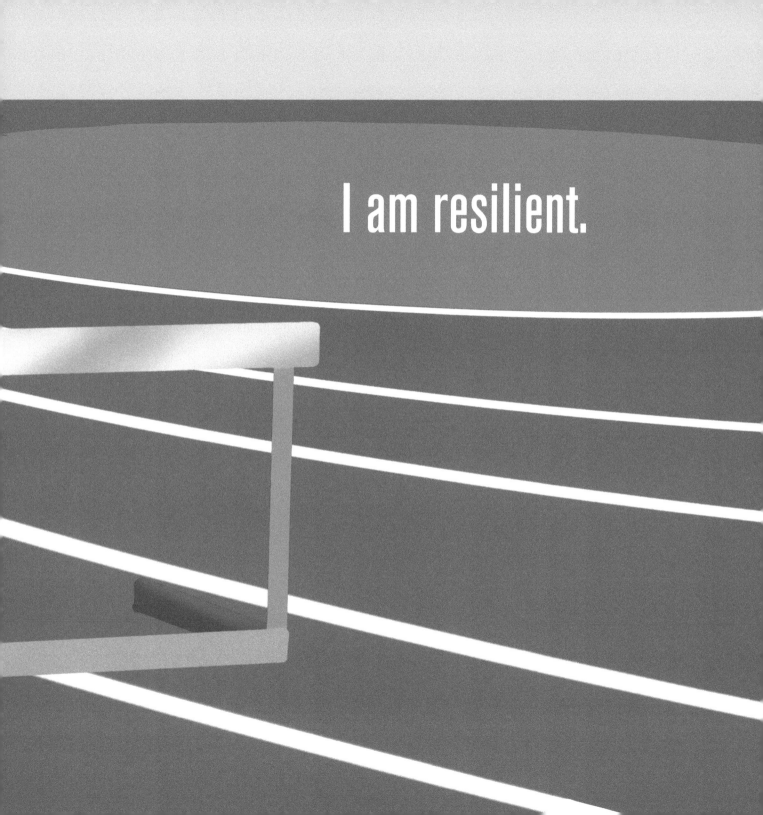

I am resilient.

# You are courageous.

You face every mountain, every challenge head on, with some help. You show up each and every day ready to do your best.

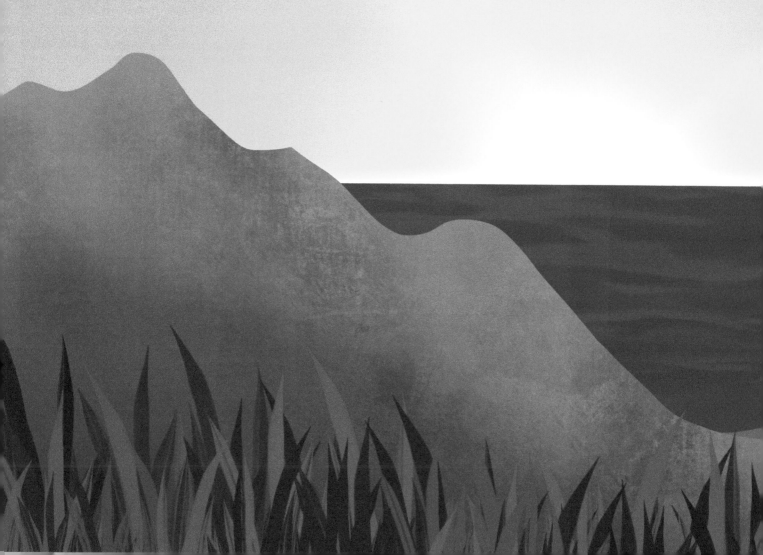

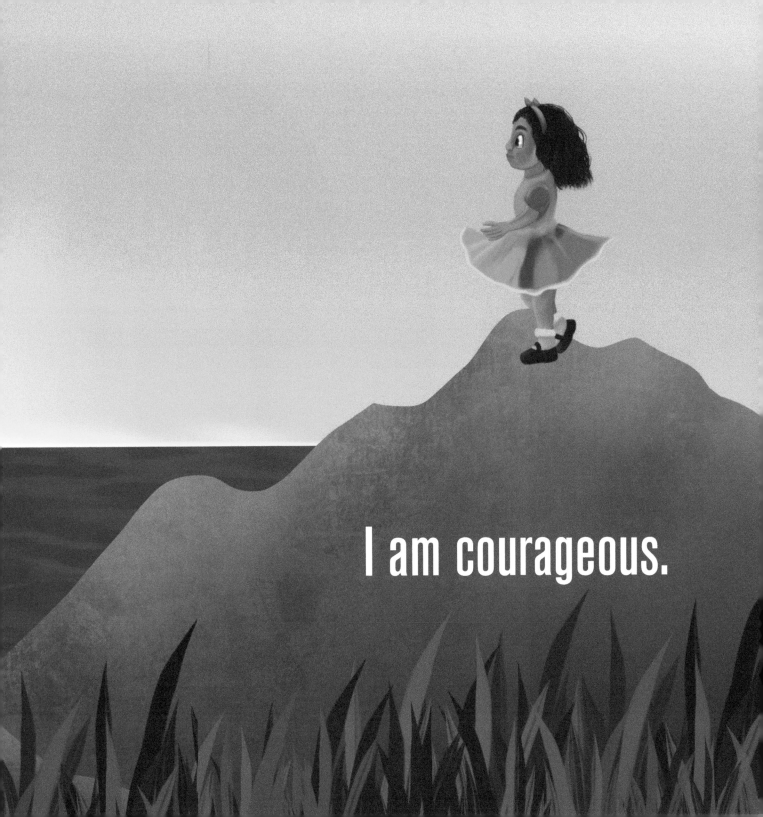

I am courageous.

# You are growing.

You know that good things take time and even though you still have ways to go, you are learning how far you have come.

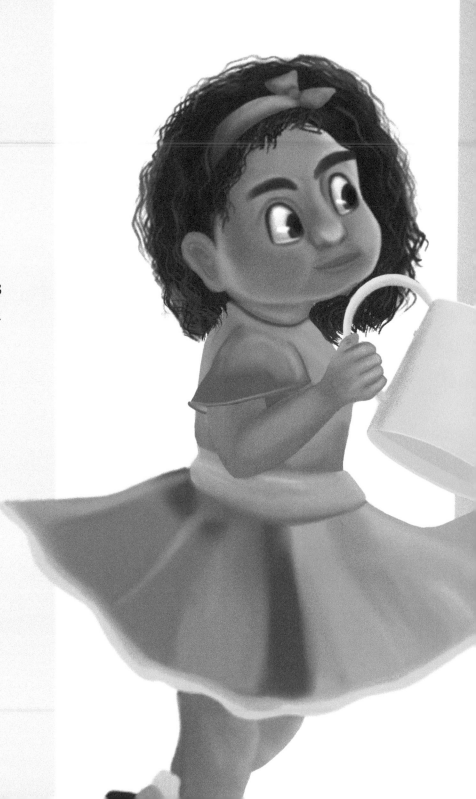

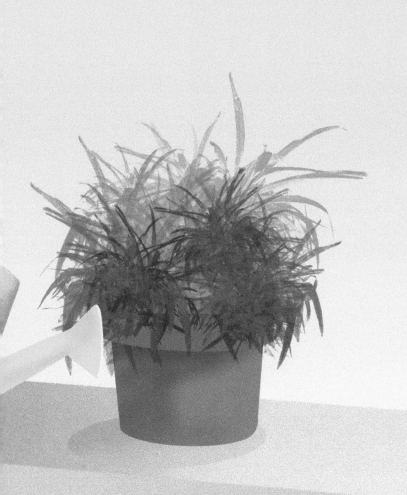

I am growing.

# You have hope.

When things did not go the way you
wanted them to, and you do not know
where tomorrow will lead, you have
hope for what lies ahead.

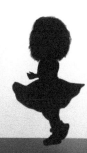

I have hope.

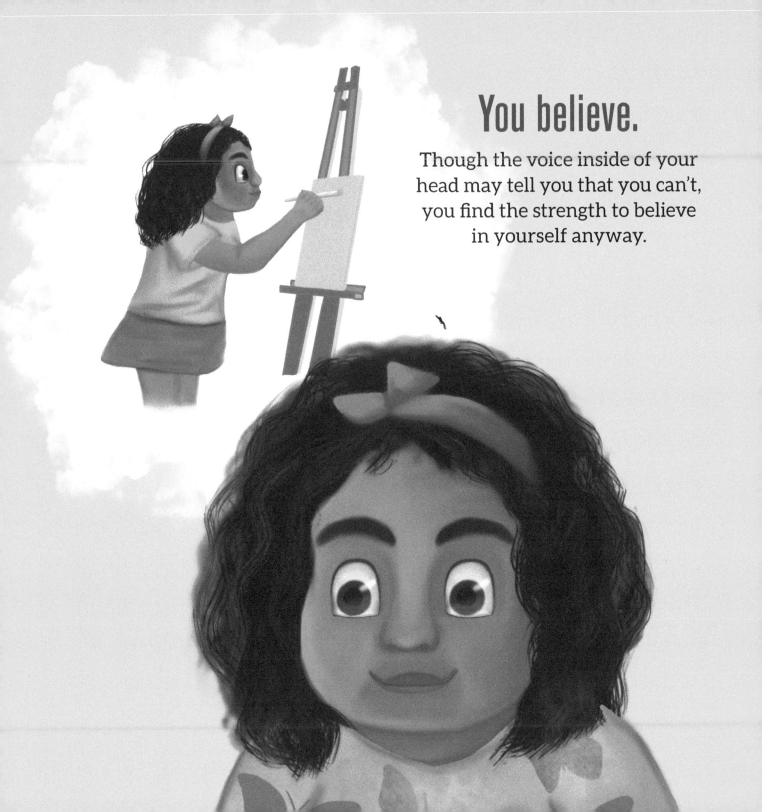

# You believe.

Though the voice inside of your head may tell you that you can't, you find the strength to believe in yourself anyway.

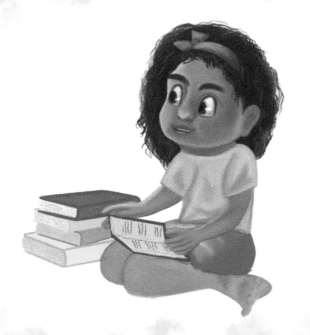

I believe.

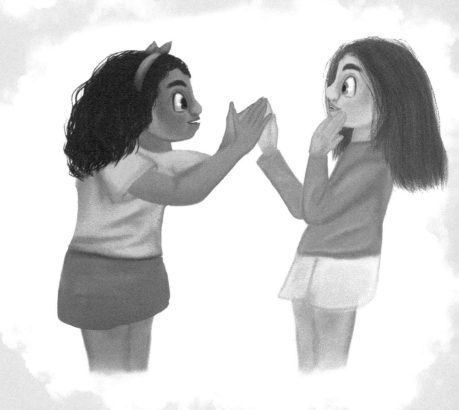

But some days you
may feel sick,

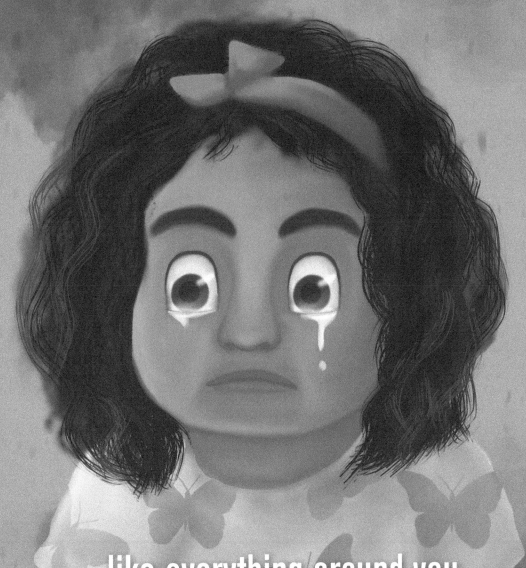
like everything around you
is grey and gloomy.

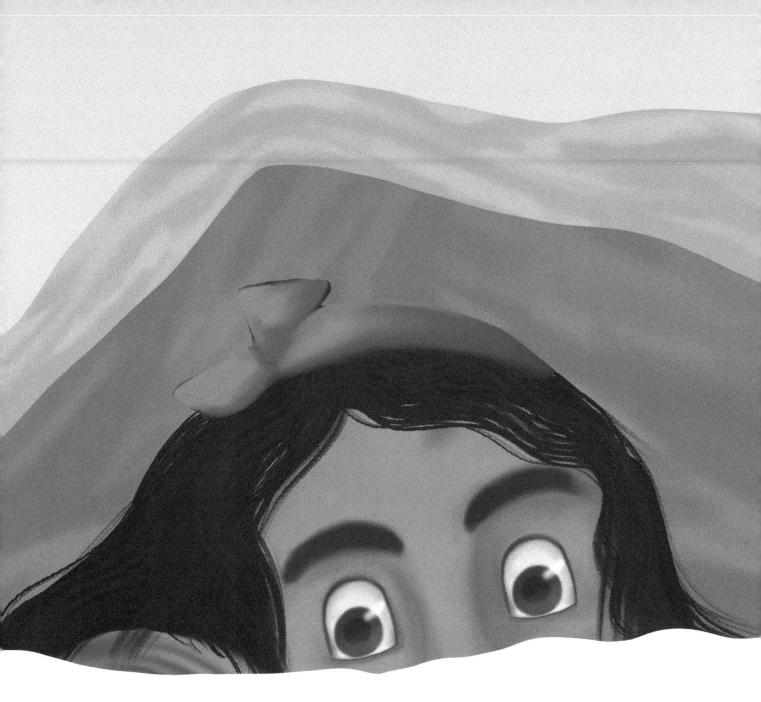

You might want to crawl back into bed and hide under the covers **until it all goes away...**

**and that's okay too.**

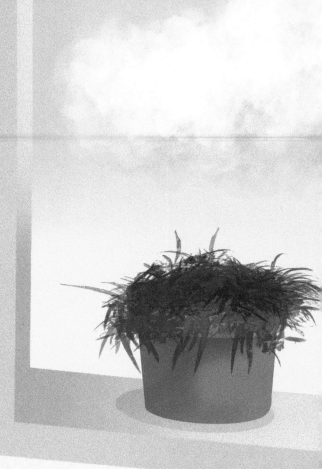
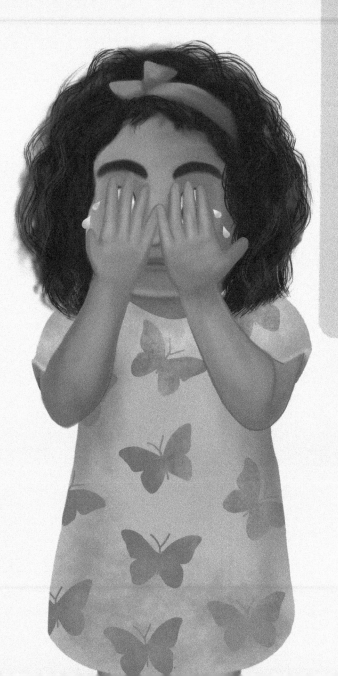

It's okay to be angry.
It's okay to be sad.
It's okay to cry.

You are more than

**where you have been.**

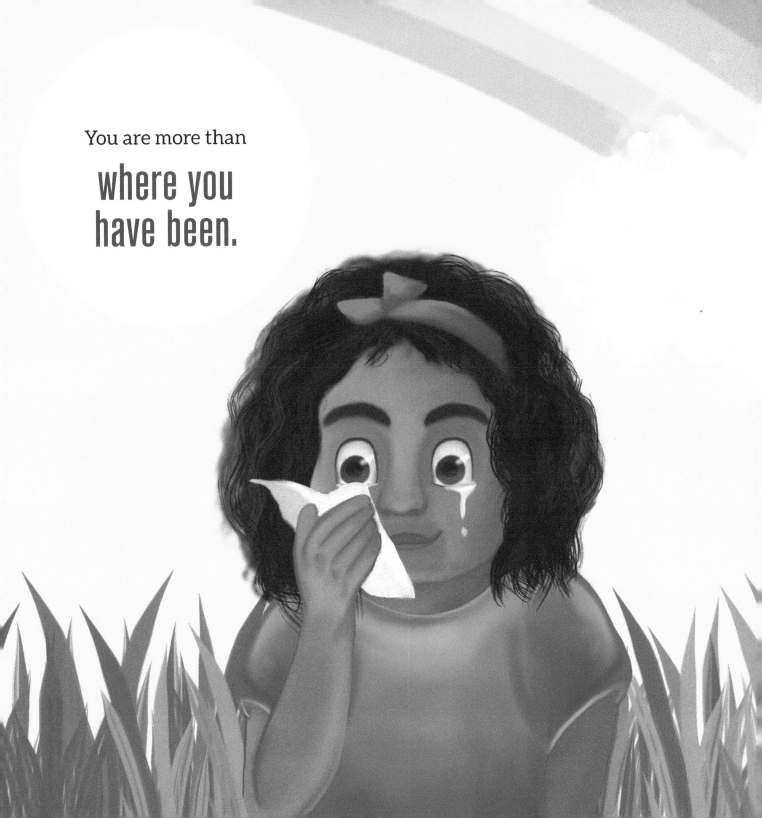

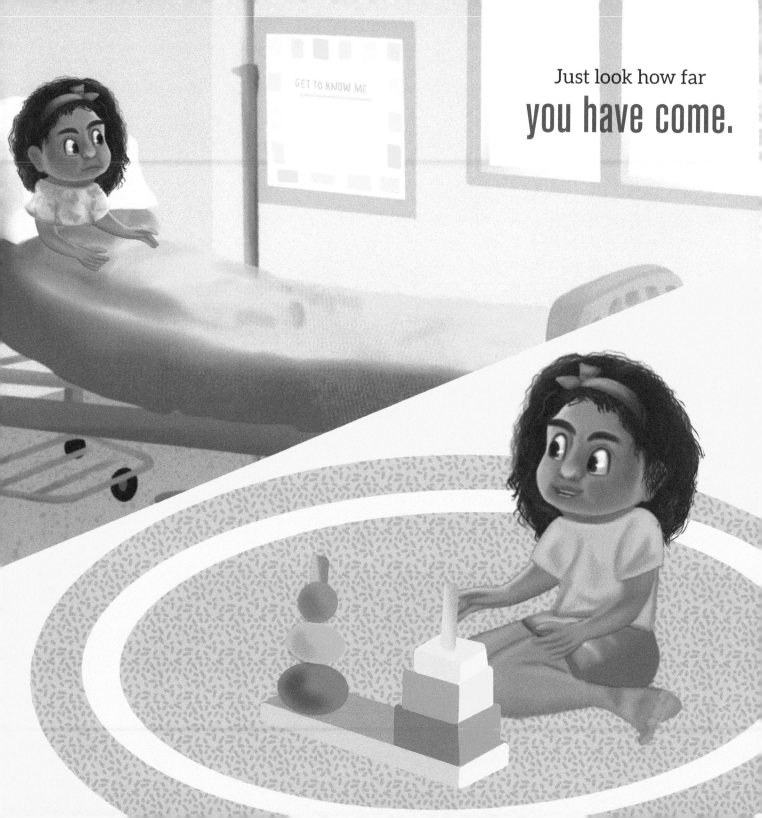

Just look how far
you have come.

# You are still the same you.

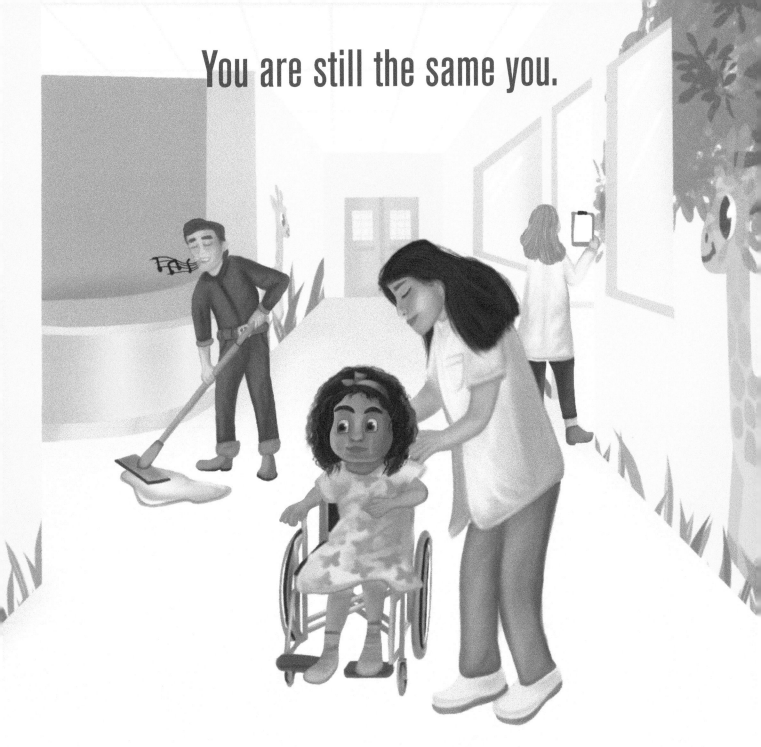

There is more to your story than what you see right here, right now.

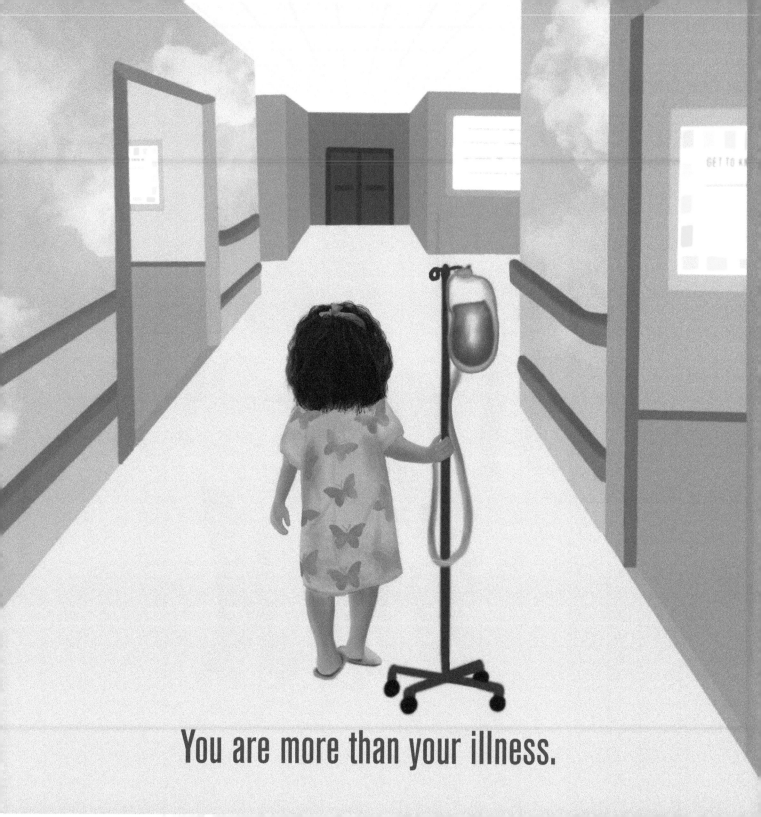

You are more than your illness.

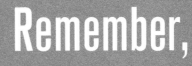

**Remember,**

there is so much more to you.

# About the Author

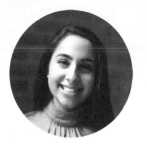

SERENA TEJPAR is a medical student at the Temerty Faculty of Medicine at the University of Toronto with a Master of Science in Global Health and a Certificate in Narrative-Based Medicine. Serena carries a passion for the intersection of health humanities and clinical practice. She was commended for her "commitment to improving the Canadian healthcare system and addressing inequities in healthcare systems worldwide" following her experience as a trauma patient after a near-fatal motor vehicle collision in 2015. She has received numerous awards and honours in recognition of her leadership, community service, and resilience including being named YMCA Ontario's Young Woman of Excellence, Top 50 Emerging Canadian Leader, and a Young Director with G(irls)20.

# About the Illustrators

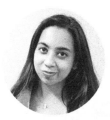

ANOOSHA LALANI is a strong proponent of storytelling as a vehicle for social activism. Her art and stories showcase minorities and cultures not often positively portrayed in the mainstream media. Having lived in Pakistan, Thailand, Indonesia, Singapore and Poland, she has had the wonderful opportunity to be exposed to a vibrant range of cultures, which have often found their way into her stories. You can find her young adult fantasy novel, *The Keepers*, at bookstores near you.

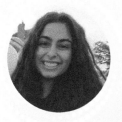

IMAN TEJPAR is currently an undergraduate student at Carleton University studying Architectural Conservation and Sustainability Engineering. Aside from her professional and academic endeavors she has a passion for fine arts and design and has recently been developing her skills in digital art. Her passion for this field also led her to illustrate her first book, *A Manual for Marco*, at the young age of 12.

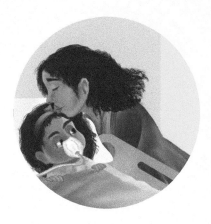

# To Parents, Caregivers, or Chosen and/or Biological Families of Children in Hospital,

It surely is not a small feat to keep strong and be fully present at all times while your child or a child you know is ill, suffering, or going through pain. What helped me as a mother with a child who was fighting for her chance at survival in the critical care unit, was keeping perspective of all that was taking place. It helped to take things one day, one moment, and one update at a time. I started each and every day with a sense of gratitude for another day. This gave me the strength to show up for my child.

It is far from easy for kids to remember to be kids when they are dealing with the challenges and emotions relating to their illness. It helps to remind them that it is okay to be upset and sad. Tears do not make them weak. Assure them that they are loved and supported no matter what happens. Remind them that WE will get through it, whatever it may be, together.

With lots of love,
Mona Kara (Serena's Mother)

# Final Word

**SHAINDY ALEXANDER**

Certified Child Life Specialist
PACT (Paediatric Advanced Care Team)
Hospital for Sick Children

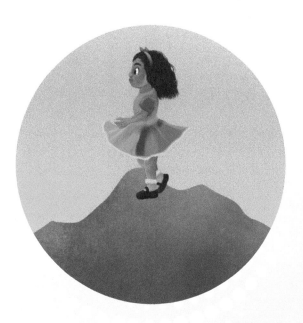

Having an illness, condition, injury, or event that impacts the health of a child can be a challenging, stressful, and often a confusing time. It is important to create a safe space for children to discuss their thoughts and emotions openly. Remember to be present, listen, validate, and feel together.

The **6C's** and **3W's** are common concerns and questions that children may have while in hospital and it is important to address these at different stages in their healthcare journey, even if your child has not brought them up themselves.

## 6 C's

*What is it CALLED?* It is important to name the condition, illness, or injury that is causing the child to be "sick". Giving the condition a name allows the child to have a greater sense of understanding and an opportunity to ask questions. Providing children with information that is honest, timely, and appropriate for their age and stage of development can help them better cope with their situation.

*Can I CATCH it?* If your child is sick with an illness that isn't contagious, reassure your child so that they do not worry about getting others sick, and share this information with other children to reassure them that they won't catch it if they share the space with the child that is ill.

*Did I CAUSE it?* Children often believe that their thoughts, behaviour, and/or wishes can influence the world around them. Although this belief is a natural part of their development, it can sometimes cause them to feel responsible for the illness. Most children wonder about what caused the illness and when they're not given the information or an explanation that is appropriate for their development and circumstance, they may feel as though they were somehow responsible. If they did have an impact on their illness or condition, remind them that sometimes things can happen that we wish didn't. It is important to allow them to talk about their feelings and concerns and feel supported and loved.

*Can I CURE it?* Children often feel a sense of responsibility to make their own illness, condition, or injury better. They may feel like they aren't doing enough or trying hard enough to get better if the treatment isn't working. Reassure them that although they can be helpful to their own treatment and/or recovery, they are not responsible for making it all better. There is a team of healthcare providers who are doing their best to help. Instead, give children jobs to help them feel included in their own healthcare journey, like taking their medicine, drawing pictures, or sharing their feelings.

*Who will take CARE of me?* When a child is in hospital, it is often common for them to worry about who will care for them and those important to them. At some point, they may believe that they are too ill to be cared for. Help your children identify adults who care about them and will help support them through this challenging time. Encourage them to ask questions and share their feelings with these people.

*How can I CONNECT to people I care about?* If children are away from their support systems and/or loved ones, remind them that there are ways to stay connected to them, including through photos, letters, phonecalls, storytelling, and connection items that they share with their loved ones. For a child who is seriously ill, share with them ways that they will always be a part of the family, even if their illness changes things.

# 3W's
## WONDER, WORRIES, and WISHES

When a child shares that they have been thinking about something challenging or scary, you may want to tell them to not WORRY and that everything will be fine, or to not cry and just stay strong. But doing so does not necessarily make the WORRIES go away. Instead, explore this thought further and discuss ways to focus on what can be controlled. Remind your child that it is okay to feel as though things are not okay, to cry, and to express their sadness or frustration. You don't need to have all the answers.

It is okay to WONDER about things, to WISH for things that may or may not be possible, and to WORRY about difficult things...together. Including them in these discussions can help children gain a sense of control, develop healthy coping skills, build trust in those around them, and increase resiliency.

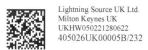

Lightning Source UK Ltd.
Milton Keynes UK
UKHW050221280622
405026UK00005B/232

9 781615 996322